One You Love Is Dying

12 Thoughts to Guide You
On the Journey

James E. Miller

Willowgreen Publishing

To John, Carrie, Martha, Chris, and Holly,
superb caregivers all

Five people deserve to claim ownership of this book. Martha Ebel, Chris Crawford, John Saynor, Holly Book, and Carrie Hackney all gave their time, their stories, their ideas, and their repeated feedback over an extended period, beginning with a delightful four-day creative session which took place in our home. Clare Barton also helped with editorial suggestions. Marty Herman did the original artwork and assisted with the design of the book. Just Sue Graphic Design executed the layout. And my wife, Bernie, did what she always does so well: she understood, she cared, and she left her own distinctive imprint throughout this work.

Willowgreen Publishing
PO Box 25180
Fort Wayne, Indiana 46825
219/424-7916

Library of Congress Catalogue
Card Number: 97-60134

ISBN 1-885933-23-1

We do not receive wisdom,
we must discover it within ourselves,
after a journey through the wilderness
which no one else can make for us,
which no one can spare us,
for our wisdom is the point of view
from which we come at last to regard the world.

MARCEL PROUST

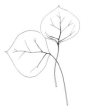

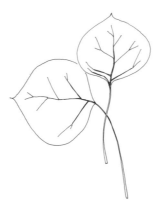

There are days when the burdens we carry
chafe our shoulders and weigh us down;
when the road seems dreary and endless,
the skies grey and threatening;
when our lives have no music in them,
and our hearts are lonely,
and our souls have lost their courage.

AUGUSTINE OF HIPPO

How often are we to die
before we go quite off this stage?
In every friend we lose,
we lose a part of ourselves,
and the best part.

ALEXANDER POPE

Someone you love is dying. It hardly seems possible. More than that, it hurts. It hurts to see them go through what they're going through. It hurts that you cannot protect them, that you cannot change the outcome. It hurts to feel all that you feel. And it hurts to realize this is not the only death you'll ever face.

Someone you love is dying and it feels as if a part of you is dying too. It's not easy to ponder what all this means. What will life be like without them? What will happen to you in the future? What will become of the relationship you've had with one another? Those are only some of your questions. You're probably also wondering about the period just ahead of you. What will you say to this person? What will you talk about? What should you not talk about? How should you act? What can you do that will best help them? And how can you best help yourself?

I've written this book to assist you in finding the answers you seek. I've made a few assumptions along the way. I've assumed you're close to the one who's dying—they're your spouse or lover, your parent or sibling or child, your close friend or trusted colleague. If your relationship is more distant, some of the specific ideas presented here may not ring true for you. The same is true if the one who's dying is very young.

I've assumed your energy level may be low and your free time limited, especially if you're already serving in a caregiving role. For that reason this book is designed to be easy to read while giving you the basic information you need. At the same time, I've assumed you may wish to reflect a bit upon all that is happening to you and to the one you care for. That's why you'll find whole pages of thoughtful quotations throughout, bringing you a sampling of accumulated wisdom going far back in time.

Not to have had pain
is not to have been human.
YIDDISH PROVERB

Heartbreak is life educating us.
GEORGE BERNARD SHAW

Suffering is a revelation.
One discovers things one never discovered before.
OSCAR WILDE

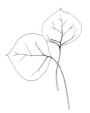

It probably will not surprise you that my interest in this topic is more than academic. I've learned what it means to be a caregiver for a seriously ill person the way you're learning—by doing it. Through the years I've also had the privilege of working cooperatively with lay and professional caregivers in many different settings. More recently I've had the wonderful opportunity to collaborate with five people, all of whom are trained professionals working daily with the dying and their caregivers. They spent several days sharing their insights and experiences with me, so this book might take the form it has taken. I am very grateful to Holly, Carrie, John, Martha, and Chris for their generous and caring counsel. I am pleased to pass along their gentle advice to you. I hope it helps. ◨

Jim Miller

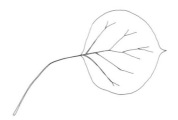

I fall upon the thorns of life.
I bleed!

PERCY BYSSHE SHELLEY

—So short a time
To teach my heart its transpositions to
This difficult and unaccustomed key!

EDNA ST. VINCENT MILLAY

1

This will be a time of testing unlike any you've known.

It is extremely stressful when someone you love is dying. Not only are you about to lose an important person, but you're probably being forced to make other major changes in your life. Change does not come easily. Unwanted change is even harder to accept. And an unwanted change which threatens your sense of well-being is the most difficult of all. It would not be surprising, then, if sometimes you feel completely overwhelmed by all this.

In addition to your emotional turmoil, you may be facing a host of disruptions in your daily life. You may be responsible for extensive caregiving duties, either ones you've chosen or ones you've been handed. Doctor's appointments, lab tests, hospital visits, and medical emergencies may devour your time. Day-to-day caregiving rituals may consume your thoughts and sap your energy. Financial matters may burden you or even frighten you. Decisions about the future may hang heavy.

Other responsibilities compete for your attention. You may have a career to juggle, other loved ones to watch over, important commitments to fulfill. Your family life may be altered, if not fractured. You probably have less leisure time and less personal privacy. If it hasn't happened already, you may have to get used to strangers in your home when medical personnel provide their specialized assistance. Friends may pull back from you out of their discomfort of not knowing what to say or do.

What is happening to the one you love may be painful to watch. Their disease may make them uncomfortable. Their treatments may make them sick. Their dying may make them very sad. You may witness changes in them that are hard to accept, or you may experience

Storms make oaks take deeper root.

GEORGE HERBERT

Pray not for lighter burdens
but for stronger backs.

THEODORE ROOSEVELT

Although the world is full of suffering,
it is also full of the overcoming of it.

HELEN KELLER

changes in your relationship that concern you, or hurt you, or mystify you.

It's no wonder that caring for someone who's dying is one of the most stress-producing jobs there is, even for people who are trained in this work. And if it so easily affects those with experience and expertise, why should it not affect you? You're new at this. And this is not just a patient you're dealing with—it's someone you love.

Your situation should not be downplayed. But neither should it be painted as impossible. Others have done what you are now called upon to do—many others. And while you may wonder if you have what it takes to do what you must do, those who have done this before you have left a message: "It's hard, but you can do it."

Three suggestions may help you through this time.

• *Learn all you can.* Find out about your loved one's disease, prognosis, and treatment. Learn how to provide care, manage stress, and develop efficiency. Ask questions, read articles and books, network with others. The more you know about what you're facing, the better you can face it.

• *Go easy on yourself.* Give yourself time to adjust to all the changes. Pace yourself daily. Be lenient in your self-expectations. The more accepting you are of yourself, the more tolerant you'll be of those around you, including the one who's so ill.

• *Don't forget: this is only temporary.* It may seem that this crisis will never end, or that life will always be sad, or that you'll be forever hurt by what's happening. But rest assured: the distress you feel will one day subside. Life's joy can return. You'll be shaped and changed by what you're going through, yet the changes don't have to be only negative. You can grow from this experience. You may not want to read that right now, but it's true.

You've known times of testing before, and you've survived them. You can yet again. For the moment draw upon the strength and the example of those who have persevered before you. Take their words to heart: "Yes, it's hard, but you can do it. You really can." ◢

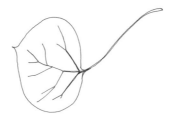

Better to be without logic than without feeling.

CHARLOTTE BRONTË

Sorrow makes us all children again.

RALPH WALDO EMERSON

*There is no way out of the desert
except through it.*

AFRICAN PROVERB

2

You'll have strong and perhaps unusual feelings, all of which deserve an outlet.

By now it's clear this experience affects you in many ways and on many levels. Consequently, it's likely you'll feel many different emotions.

The most common response is sorrow. It can be unspeakably sad to care for someone you're close to as they go through the dying process. You may feel as if your heart will break, seeing what's happening to them, knowing what's happening to you. Some days you may feel afraid, wondering what lies in store for each of you and all of you. You may feel anxious sometimes, worried other times.

You may feel guilty for things you've done or not done, either through the years or only yesterday. Some caregivers feel guilty for disliking some of the tasks they must perform, or for being healthy when the other is so ill, or for wanting this time to be over with, or for living on when the other is dying. You may feel helpless, unable to change these circumstances or to help the other person feel any better.

A feeling which may surprise you is your anger. You may be mad all this is happening to the one you love, and to you too. *"It's not fair!"* you may say. *"We don't deserve this!"* you may cry. You may find yourself getting mad at doctors and nurses, or at friends who avoid you, or at drivers who go too fast, or at elevators that go too slow. Those nearest to you may receive your ire—family members perhaps, or the one who is dying, especially if they have also been angry at you. You may feel resentful, sometimes being irritated about the extra work you must do, or the sacrifices you must make, or the appreciation you must forgo.

I sometimes hold it half a sin
To put in words the grief I feel;
For words, like Nature, half reveal
And half conceal the Soul within.

ALFRED, LORD TENNYSON

Who never broke with tears, his bread,
Who never watched through anguished hours
With weeping eyes, upon his bed,
He knows ye not, O heavenly Powers.

JOHANN WOLFGANG VON GOETHE

Your main feeling may be confusion—that often happens. It's not uncommon to feel numb, like you're in shock, especially early on. You may feel bored, because caregiving has its tedious moments.

You may have positive feelings as well—affection for the one you're caring for, respect for what they've done and what they're doing, joy for what you can celebrate and share, perhaps wonder for the gifts you receive when you least expect them. You may feel proud for many different reasons, or grateful for no reason at all other than the fact you have been given this day and it is good.

Caregivers often find their emotions contradict one another. You may experience unpredictable mood swings which can lead you to wonder about your own stability or even your sanity. If this is happening to you, rest assured you're not unusual. This is a strange time in your life, and strange feelings may well occur. Indeed, if you had only ordinary feelings at such an extraordinary time, wouldn't that be strange?

Whatever you feel, find ways to express it. If you bury your feelings, you'll spend precious energy trying to *keep* them buried, energy you could put to good use in more productive ways. And the truth is, you *can't* keep your feelings buried entirely. Whether you recognize it or not, they'll come out in other ways. So find at least one person you can talk with regularly. Better yet, find more than one. Write about your feelings in letters or a journal. If it's your style, express yourself with music or art. Make something with your hands or do something with your whole body. Cry your feelings, or pray them.

Don't ignore your feelings. Recognize them. Accept them. Value them. They're a sign of your humanness and that's where your strength as a caregiver lies. ◪

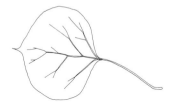

I think character never changes;
the acorn becomes an oak,
which is very little like an acorn to be sure,
but it never becomes an ash.
HESTER LYNCH PIOZZI

To be what we are,
and to become what we are capable of becoming,
is the only end of life.
ROBERT LOUIS STEVENSON

3

The dying person will be as they've always been, only more so.

When someone is told they have only limited time to live, they respond in their own unique way. Some people become visibly upset and others appear stoic. Some act astonished and others take it in stride, as if they've known all along. Some reach out to those around and others withdraw into themselves. There are no prescriptions for how people will react when they learn they're dying, but there are some general rules.

• *As a rule, the kind of person they've been before is the kind of person they'll be now.*

The fact that someone is now dying does not change who they are. They do not automatically become wiser or kinder or braver. They simply become more themselves. Generally, if they were serious before, they'll be serious now. If they've been lighthearted, they'll probably still have a sparkle about them, at least some of the time. Quiet people will usually not talk a lot more, grouchy people will not complain much less, and affectionate people will not give up their loving ways.

What dying people may do is emphasize certain aspects of who they've been all along. Realizing this is a time unlike any other, and knowing it will not come again, they may concentrate on certain pursuits or call upon certain characteristics, letting others fall away. You may have the impression they're becoming more who they're meant to be.

• *As a rule, dying people prefer to live fully as long as they're able and to be treated as very much alive.*

There's a tendency to treat dying people differently. Voices are often lowered. People's faces may appear overly somber or take on a

Trust thyself:
every heart vibrates to that iron string.
RALPH WALDO EMERSON

The snow goose need not bathe
to make itself white.
Neither need you do anything
but be yourself.
LAO-TSE

false cheeriness. Topics of conversation become more limited and some things are no longer talked about at all. As a result, the dying person may feel they're being pushed to one side, or they're being treated with pity, or they're being handled like a child.

Not only is the dying person no different than they used to be, but in the most essential way, they are no different than you are today. They're your equal in every sense. They're as full of life as you are. They're every bit as human and maybe even *more* human. So they may bristle if you treat them as less than they are. They don't want your pity; they want your compassion. They don't want you to pat them on the head; they want you to go with them hand-in-hand just as far as you can.

• *As a rule, rules don't always hold.*

While most people don't experience personality conversions as they prepare to die, some do. Some decide to live the time that's left in radically different ways, and they give up old ways of being for new ones. Some become obviously freer and others become clearly happier. Some grow up a great deal in a short period of time and a few, unlikely as it may seem, actually blossom. It happens.

It will help everyone if you can go into this experience with as few preconceptions as possible about what dying people are like. Expect the one you love to live as fully as they want for as long as they're able. Expect them to know joy as well as sorrow, to feel promise as well as pain, to laugh as well as cry. Expect them to teach you what you need to know. Mostly, just expect them to live until they die. Then let them do precisely that. ◼

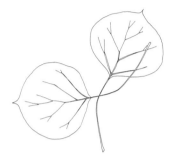

It is difficult for one person to act a play.
CHINESE PROVERB

Be patient with everyone,
but above all with yourself.
ST. FRANCIS DE SALES

We cannot do everything at once,
but we can do something at once.
CALVIN COOLIDGE

4

You cannot do everything yourself.

If you're the primary caregiver of one who's dying, this is likely to be the most exhausting thing you've ever done. Your workload is enormous. The pressures upon you are huge. Your needs are many. No matter how skilled or strong or experienced you are, you cannot do it all. Some tasks are too technical, some too physically demanding, some too emotionally draining. You need others to help you with the load.

• *Let others share the load for your sake.* Everyone has limits. Acknowledging yours is not a sign of weakness but an indication of wisdom and maturity. It shows you know yourself and you understand the complexity of what must be done. When help is offered, accept it. And when someone says, "Let me know if there's anything I can do," take them at their word and let them know. Be specific. People can help you by cooking meals, doing household chores, shopping, and picking up medical supplies. They can care for the one who's ill while you're away, sit with them while you're otherwise engaged, escort you or them on trips to the doctor, or serve as your link to the outside world by taking and making telephone calls. Knowledgeable individuals can help you make financial decisions, or find spiritual support, or get your legal affairs in order.

What if help is not offered? Ask for it. Tell family and friends what you need. Let professionals know what would help. Seek out support services and volunteer agencies. If you haven't already, contact your local hospice. They have loads of information and unequaled expert care—no one can help you more.

• *Let others share the load for their sake.* You're not the only one who benefits when help is provided. Your helpers also benefit. Often they're eager to demonstrate their concern and love, and they feel

Such ever was love's way:
to rise, it stoops.
ROBERT BROWNING

The hands that help are holier
than the lips that pray.
ROBERT INGERSOLL

Such help as we can give to each other in this world
is a debt to each other.
JOHN RUSKIN

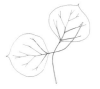

deprived if they cannot. When they have certain tasks to perform, their visits can be more natural, for they have a contribution to make, a subject to talk about, and perhaps a reason to return. Like everyone in this drama, your helpers feel powerless too. Having something to do is one way they can grapple with not being able to do more.

• *Let others share the load for the sake of the dying person.* It helps the one at the center of these events to realize how much she or he matters to others. They appreciate knowing that you are being supported too, and that whatever burden is unavoidably created, it's being spread among many. When other caregivers are involved, it can add variety and spice to the dying person's days. It can help assure them of the best possible care, since you can be more comfortable in your primary role, and more relaxed, and more refreshed.

• *Let others share the load for the sake of the common good.* Years ago neighbors used to come together to help a family with a barn raising and within a day or two the job would be done—a feat much too big for a single individual or even a small group. Generations had fun together, human bonds were reinforced, and important work was done at the same time. Something similar can happen when people work together as a team to offer care. The meaning of family is expanded, the sense of community is affirmed and brought to life, and wonderful work is done simultaneously. The example of cooperative caring you help develop today can become a model for others tomorrow. It is a model our world is waiting for.

Of all the reasons to seek and accept help as you care for the one you love, none is more important than this: you deserve it, all of you. ◨

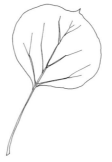

Self-sacrifice is a thing
which should be put down by law.
It is so demoralizing to the people
for whom one sacrifices oneself.

OSCAR WILDE

But how shall we expect charity toward others,
when we are uncharitable to ourselves?
Charity begins at home.

THOMAS BROWNE

5

To be a good caregiver, you must take good care of yourself.

You may not realize how much your health can be jeopardized when you're a primary caregiver. You may not eat as well as you should or sleep as well as you could. You may become physically, emotionally, or spiritually depleted. You will be grieving about what's happening and what will yet happen, draining your inner resources still more. Caregivers sometimes express their dilemma this way: "I feel so weak, yet I must act so strong." Perhaps that's how you feel.

In such a chaotic time, what can you do to make things go as well as possible? You can make sure you take care of yourself. After all, if you don't stay fit, you can't provide the kind of healthy caregiving you wish and the other person requires.

• *Honor your physical needs.* Your body cannot keep up with the demands of caring for another unless you help it. Eat balanced meals. Take vitamin supplements. Give yourself plenty of rest breaks. Find ways to get the sleep you need. Exercise regularly. Watch carefully any self-medications, whatever form those may take. Learn and practice relaxation techniques. Treat your body as a partner in this venture, not a slave.

• *Cultivate efficiency.* Do what's necessary, then let the little things slide. Develop shortcuts in your chores. Learn to organize meals, errands, and schedules to save time and preserve energy. Allow others to assist you in being even more efficient.

• *Set your boundaries.* Remember you deserve time and space for yourself. Remember you have a right to your own feelings, whatever they are, and you don't have to take on the feelings of others. Remember you don't have to live up to other people's expectations,

What is life if, full of care,
We have no time to stand and stare?

WILLIAM HENRY DAVIES

You may have to live in a crowd,
but you do not have to live like it,
nor subsist on its food.
You may have your own orchard.
You may drink at a hidden spring.
Be yourself if you would serve others.

HENRY VAN DYKE

especially when those don't feel right. In other words, remember that "No" is a complete sentence. So is "I don't want to."

• *Maintain some normalcy.* As much as you're able, keep doing those activities you've always enjoyed. Maintain some of your everyday routines, especially if you have a family at home. Stay in touch with friends. Remain involved with life in those ways that nourish your mind, heart, and soul.

• *Take time away.* This may be difficult to do when you're so concerned about the one who is ill, but it's important. Do those things that give you a break and refresh you—see a movie, dine with a friend, get a massage, walk in nature. Participate in those things that bring you pleasure, however small. Or, if you want, just do nothing at all for awhile.

• *Make room for humor.* There are reasons to smile, even at times like this. Make your own reasons if you must. Watch funny movies or TV comedies. Joke with one another. Recount humorous events from the past. Whether you giggle or guffaw, do it out loud.

• *Detach from results.* You may wish for something specific to happen as a result of what you do—a sign of improvement, an expression of gratitude, a change of mood. However hard you work, such results are beyond your control. So do what seems natural and right, then let go of the consequences which may or may not follow. Don't let the value of your caregiving depend upon how someone else responds.

• *Stay in the moment.* Focus on each day, one at a time. Avoid looking too far forward. Concentrate on what the present offers. Be deliberate in what you're doing, how you're doing it, and why you're doing it. Breathe in your satisfactions. Breathe out your disappointments. Linger over traces of beauty. Savor happinesses. Live.

You don't know how long this journey you're on will last. You must marshal your reserves for what lies ahead. So help everyone by taking extremely good care of yourself. ◪

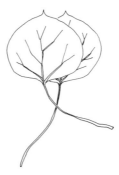

Respect yourself and others will respect you.

CONFUCIUS

One can never consent to creep
when one feels an impulse to soar.

HELEN KELLER

Thy purpose firm is equal to the deed;
Who does the best his circumstance allows
Does well, acts nobly; angels could do no more.

EDWARD YOUNG

6

The one who's dying is in charge.

You and the dying person have an equality to your relationship—
you both have something to give and you each have something to
receive. But in one fundamental way you're not equal: the person
who is dying gets to make certain important decisions on their own.
And some of those decisions may impact you.

It's as if a drama were being played out before everyone's eyes. In
that drama there's only one leading character; everyone else has a
supporting role. The person at center stage is the one whose life is
drawing to a close. He or she merits the attention and the authori-
ty that goes with that part.

The dying person has needs to be met and rights to be acknowl-
edged. Obviously, they're the one most deeply affected by their illness. They're the only one who can know what this experience is like
for them—any fear or pain, any dread or embarrassment, any despair
or loneliness. In light of what's happening to them, they're entitled
to be as comfortable as possible. They deserve to be listened to carefully and treated respectfully. They deserve to keep whatever power
is rightfully theirs.

They should have their say about their home environment.
Which room will be theirs and where will their bed be? What light-
ing would they like? Will there be music, and if so, what kind? Will
there be pictures? Flowers? Reading material? Pets? Will people be
around? Who? When? For how long? As much as possible, the dying
person should be the one to decide.

The one who's dying should also play the central role on their
medical team. They have the right to be informed about their disease
and prognosis, if they wish to be. It's their right to make decisions
about who provides their medical care, the kind of care they're given,

Where we are free to act,
we are also free to refrain from acting,
and where we are able to say "No,"
we are also able to say "Yes."

ARISTOTLE

If a man does not keep pace with his companions,
perhaps it is because he hears a different drummer.
Let him step to the music he hears,
however measured or far away.

HENRY DAVID THOREAU

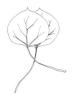

and where that care is given. They may turn to others for feedback and advice, but they should not be required to live with decisions made by others which do not take into account their own best interests, their physical comfort, and their peace of mind. The one who is dying may make decisions you do not like, creating pain for both of you. Ultimately, however, theirs is the voice to be heard above all others.

Of course, they are not to inflict harm on themselves or other people. They are not to deny you your rights or to expect you to compromise your own health. They are not to try to manipulate your feelings. Should that happen, you will need to stand up for what is right for you.

The time will come when this drama will begin to shift. The dying person's ability to make decisions will decline. But until that happens, your role as a caregiver is to encourage, support, and carry out the decisions they make. You are not to act for them without their agreement. You are not to speak for them without their permission. And you are not to think for them unless they can no longer think for themselves.

This is their show. Let them be the star. ◪

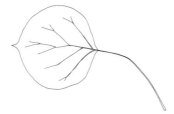

What do we live for
if not to make life less difficult for each other?
GEORGE ELIOT (MARY ANN EVANS)

Love consists in this,
that two solitudes protect and touch
and greet each other.
RAINER MARIA RILKE

Talking is like playing on the harp;
there is as much in laying the hands
on the strings to stop their vibration
as in twanging them to bring out their music.
OLIVER WENDELL HOLMES

7

The one who's dying needs you to reach out.

Those who know they're dying may hesitate to voice their deepest thoughts and feelings. They're often afraid of upsetting people around them. They're not sure how much others are ready for. It's not unusual for caregivers to behave similarly, tiptoeing carefully through conversations, steering clear of any topics that might seem disturbing. This can also be a way of protecting oneself. Whatever the reason, the result is the same: the dying person can come to feel isolated and lonely. So can you. But that doesn't have to be the case. You can reach out and connect.

• *Connect by talking.* Speak to the one you care for as an equal, person to person, face to face. Say what you think. Express what you feel. If the dying person is slow to open up, don't push them. Just let them know you're ready to move to a deeper level whenever they are. If tears come, let them be. They're a sign that you care, an indication you wish this wasn't happening. Would you want the one you're with to think otherwise? Be honest with them. Talk simply and straightforwardly. Avoid secrets. Speak when the time is right and stop when the moment has passed. Draw the other person out bit by bit. Allow yourself to be drawn out too. Make this a time when you truly meet.

• *Connect by listening.* The one who's dying may have much to say—feelings to explore, questions to ask, experiences to sum up, ideas to leave behind. Your patient, attentive ear is one of the greatest gifts you can offer. Real listening takes work. The dying person's thoughts can be complicated and confusing as they spill out. Their emotions can be forceful and yet elusive. Answers may be hard to come by. Yet you will perform a wonderful service by listening care-

When a companion's heart of itself overflows,
the best one can do is to do nothing.

HERMAN MELVILLE

We can make our minds so like still water
that beings gather about us,
that they may see their own images,
and so live for a moment with a clearer,
perhaps even with a fiercer, life
because of our quiet.

WILLIAM BUTLER YEATS

fully to what the other person has to say, without interrupting, judging, or shying away. These can be sacred times you'll remember long afterward.

• *Connect by encouraging memories.* Often a dying person wants to make sense of their time on earth. They want to feel their life has mattered and their influence will not be forgotten. You can play a critical role by treating their memories as important and their reflections on life as valuable. Leaf through scrapbooks and old letters with them. Look at pictures, sort through mementos, tell and re-tell meaningful stories. As you do this, you're each beginning to say your goodbyes. Saying them this way, gradually and lovingly, can help you both.

• *Connect by touching.* People who are dying want to know you're with them in as many ways as possible. No way is more direct than physical touch. If it's a comfort to them, hold their hand or touch their arm or shoulder or head. Stroke them, massage them, hug them. Your nonverbal communication can say as much as your verbal, or even more. Remember that touch and hearing are the two senses a person retains longest. Even when they cannot speak, they can be spoken to with a gentle caress or soothing words.

• *Connect by just being present.* Sometimes the most thoughtful way to reach out to a dying person is by not saying or doing anything. By your consistent return you communicate "I will not desert you." By sitting or working quietly in the same room, you communicate "I enjoy being with you." By staying beside them when they need you, your message is clear: "I am right here. I care."

The one who is dying wants to know they're not alone. It's up to you to tell them in as many ways as you can. ◪

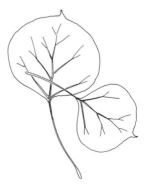

All things must change to something new,
to something strange.

HENRY WADSWORTH LONGFELLOW

Wherever we are,
it is but a stage on the way to somewhere else,
and whatever we do,
however well we do it,
it is only preparation to do something else
that shall be different.

ROBERT LOUIS STEVENSON

8

Your relationship will change as you go.

Because the two of you share a bond that's unique, it's impossible to predict exactly what will happen to your relationship as the days unfold. It's unlikely, however, that it will remain the same. Too much will be changing around you for a change not to occur between you.

• *A special closeness may develop.* When it becomes clear the time you'll have together is limited, you may go to a deeper level in your relationship than you ordinarily would. You may choose to address problems that have separated you. You may speak words of appreciation or love you haven't spoken in a long time, or perhaps ever. You may come to new understandings of one another, new ways of being with one another. Your present experience may unite you as you've never been united.

That doesn't mean you won't have conflicts. That can easily happen during times of high stress and strong feelings. But these very disagreements can be opportunities for both of you—you can become more forgiving, more understanding, more genuine with one another. Sometimes, unfortunately, individuals and families cannot bridge their differences and they become more estranged from one another. If this is happening, perhaps a counselor or other caring professional can help you re-establish ties before it's too late.

• *In time the dying person will probably depend on you more.* While it's important not to take from them their power or freedom, the one who's dying may come to count on you in ways they have not in the past. They may require more physical assistance or emotional support. They may look to you for help in their planning or with their thinking. They may ask you to take over for them in vari-

All things change, nothing is extinguished.
OVID

My boat goes west, yours east
heaven's a wind for both journeys.
CHAO LI-HUA

Love is the only thing
we can carry with us when we go,
and it makes the end so easy.
LOUISA MAY ALCOTT

ous ways. This may be hard for you to do, but it's another of those challenges your caregiving may require.

• *Eventually the dying person will begin to withdraw.* The time will come when they will start to turn inward and pull back from the external world. They'll want to see fewer people. They'll desire more quietness. You may find it especially difficult when they start to retreat from you. You may feel it's a negation of your relationship, but it's not that at all. It's a part of the great mystery of dying. They are not withdrawing from you so much as from life itself.

It will help you both if you can unhook yourself from feelings of rejection. They know you cannot go where they're going and they're simply doing what they must. As they withdraw, they may turn to another person to help them—a professional caregiver perhaps, or someone who has been with other people as they neared death. You may want to turn to another person to help you through this time too.

• *The one who's dying will want to know you're with them to the end.* Even as they pull away, they will want to feel they're cared for and they have your blessing to go. It may help them to hear those very words. It may also help you to say them. They will be able to sense you're with them when you whisper your love, when you promise your remembrance, when you hold them with tenderness, when you honor them with tears.

As the end approaches, your relationship will shift. But that will not take away from the bond you've had before, nor will it limit the bond you'll have afterwards. ◼

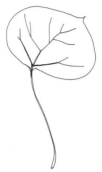

If one does not decide when one should,
someone will suffer the consequences.

CHINESE PROVERB

When you have to make a choice
and don't make it,
that is in itself a choice.

WILLIAM JAMES

The greatest firmness is the greatest mercy.

HENRY WADSWORTH LONGFELLOW

9

Making important decisions early can head off significant problems later.

As someone's life comes to an end, decisions must be made which can affect many people. Ideally, the dying person will do this on their own or in collaboration with others. These end-of-life matters cannot be passed over. If the dying person does not attend to them, someone else will have to. That "someone" may be you.

It's neither fair nor wise to rush the dying individual to make these decisions too quickly. It takes time to adjust to the reality of all that's happening and will yet happen. These decisions require both thought and energy, and this is a time when charged emotions can complicate the process. Yet it makes sense to handle these matters early, while various options still exist, while their thinking is still clear, and before others are forced to make decisions for them without adequate information.

• *Certain decisions will influence how they live and die.* Nowadays human life can be sustained for long periods, whether or not the person is conscious, whether or not that's what they want. In executing *advance medical directives,* including what's often called a *living will,* a person spells out their wishes about what will and will not be done to them in the event of medical crisis. Other documents can be drawn up which name who will make various medical and legal decisions when the dying person is no longer able to do so. It's important to consult an attorney who understands the laws where you live.

The one who's dying may want to clarify their thoughts about how they'll spend the last part of their life—what they'll do and not do, who'll be present and who won't, where they'll choose to pass their time, both early on and later. Do they prefer home care or insti-

Only stay quiet while my mind remembers
The beauty of fire from the beauty of embers.
JOHN MASEFIELD

At the going down of the sun and in the morning
We shall remember them.
LAURENCE BINYON

When eating a fruit,
think of the person who planted the tree.
VIETNAMESE PROVERB

tutional care? Who will be on their caregiving team? If choice is possible, where would they like to die?

• *Certain decisions will apply to the time right after they die.* Will there be a burial, a cremation, or will their body be donated to science? What do they wish their funeral or memorial service to be like? Where and when will it take place? Who will speak? Are there readings they particularly desire? Certain music? Special requests about the way they're remembered or their life is celebrated? Thoughts like these may seem overwhelming for you at the moment. Give yourself time; you'll get used to them. You, the dying person, or both of you may wish to consult with a funeral director in advance. These professionals can be a real help.

• *Other decisions involve the longer period after their death.* Certainly a will should be prepared, giving instructions about one's assets and family matters. When the time is right, plans should be made for the distribution of their personal effects, as well as special gifts they wish to make. Naming an executor to oversee these matters will smooth and simplify the process.

Remember it helps the dying person to communicate their final wishes. It gives them a certain amount of control. It can bring them peace of mind. It can help them do their own grief work. And it can offer them ways to leave their legacy.

Of course, all this will help you too. You can have the satisfaction of knowing you're carrying out your loved one's requests. You can sidestep problems which might develop from any painful or unpopular decisions you had to make in the absence of their input. You can be freed to do what is yours—to provide the best care you can while they're living, to put in place the most appropriate commemoration at their death, and then to live from that moment on as fully as you can as a loving, grieving, healing person. ◪

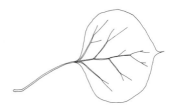

I put forward formless and unresolved notions...
not to establish the truth but to seek it.
MICHEL DE MONTAIGNE

Do we decide questions at all?
We decide answers, no doubt;
but surely the questions decide us.
LEWIS CARROLL

What are heavy? Sea-sand and sorrow;
What are brief? Today and tomorrow;
What are frail? Spring blossoms and youth;
What are deep? The ocean and truth.
CHRISTINA ROSSETTI

10

This is a natural time for inner searching.

People who know they're dying often become more reflective. Sometimes they pose questions that are hard, if not impossible, to answer. They may worry about what will happen after they die. They may talk about spiritual matters more than they ever have. They may have unusual spiritual experiences they'll want to share with you. Of course, the dying person is not the only one who'll undertake this inner search. Chances are you will too.

• *You will be confronted with life's difficult questions.* "Why do they have this disease?" you may ask. "Why can't something more be done?" If they're in pain, you may question why they suffer. If their death seems untimely, you may wonder why they're being punished unfairly. You may ask similar questions about yourself, knowing your own pain is different, but it's no less real. "Why them?" you may plead. "Why us? Why now?" It's healthy to allow your thoughts and questions to surface, because they're natural ones. And it's not unreasonable nor is it sinful to raise issues like these, even if it means raising them to God. Your honest questions should not be stifled. They should be honored for what they are—your serious attempts to arrive at the truth.

• *You stand before life's remarkable mysteries.* The person you care for will soon cross a barrier you cannot, yet a barrier you will some day cross yourself. What lies on the other side? For all the predictions and promises, it remains a mystery. While death is perhaps life's *greatest* mystery, it's not the *only* mystery. No sooner do you ask "What is death?" than you're faced with other questions: "What is life? Where does it come from? Where does it go?" If you ask "Why this illness?", what about also asking "Why so much health *before*

*One cannot help but be in awe
when he contemplates the mysteries of eternity,
of life, of the marvelous structure of reality.
It is enough if one tries merely
to comprehend a little of this mystery every day.
Never lose a holy curiosity.*

ALBERT EINSTEIN

*There aren't many mysteries,
but there is one upon which everything depends,
and it is so immense that it fills the whole space.*

CARLO CARRETTO

*Your lamp was lit from another lamp.
All God wants is your gratitude for that.*

RUMI

this illness?" And this: "Why can psychological and spiritual healing take place even when there's no prospect of physical healing?" In addition to "Why this sadness?", what about "Why this love we feel? Why the joy that sometimes breaks through? Why all the blessings we've been given in the past and are ours yet today?" It's all quite a mystery, isn't it?

• *You may find yourself in the midst of the Eternal Mystery.* As you care for someone who's dying, you may sense there's more to this experience than what the two of you bring. In addition to your presence, you may discover God's presence. In addition to what *you* do, you may realize something is being done *through* you and *in* you and *around* you, and it's ever so much greater than you. A sense of sacredness often settles over a time of dying. A sanctity can envelop your caregiving. When you try to describe it, words fail. If that's your experience, let it be. Words aren't necessary—in fact, they may only get in the way.

Make room for your spirituality as a caregiver. Find a "soul friend" and talk. Keep a journal of your dreams and prayers. Carve out a quiet time each day and meditate. Listen to music that inspires you. If you're so inclined, turn to the resources of your faith—read scriptures, pray, commune, worship. Let this period of your life be what it will be for you spiritually. And that means it may not be a spiritual time for you. Some find their inner search does not begin until later, when their caregiving responsibilities are behind them. You'll figure out what's right for you. Just be sure to seek your own answers, not someone else's. ◪

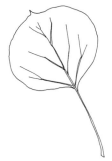

*A man's dying is more the survivor's affair
than his own.*

THOMAS MANN

God prepares the cure before the hurt.

THE TALMUD

*He who lacks time to mourn
lacks time to mend.*

WILLIAM SHAKESPEARE

11

This experience will extend beyond the end of your caregiving.

Your work as a caregiver may seem unending. Weeks may turn into months, and those months into a year or two or more. If you're resourceful, you'll find ways to pace yourself, knowing the time just before a person dies can be especially exhausting. If you're fortunate, you'll find the support you need all along the way so you can maintain your reserves. And if you're wise, you won't fall into the trap of anticipating that when your caregiving stops, the most painful part will be over. Perhaps it will be. Perhaps it won't.

No one knows what you'll feel or how you'll behave when the one you love dies. You're much too original for that. But whenever it happens, you *will* have a response. And however you respond, it will be a continuation of what is happening to you now.

If there is one truth that holds, it is this: *Even if you think you're ready for the person to die, you're never quite ready for them to die.* Even if it's not a surprise, even if your farewells have been said, even if it finally seems all for the best, it's still a shock. It still requires adjustment. It still hurts.

There is a related truth: *Even if you've grieved your loss before they die, you must still grieve your loss after they die.* However conscientiously and openly you've done your grieving beforehand, you have another dimension of grief to experience once you can no longer see them or talk to them in person. You can prepare yourself for this later time, but you cannot shortcut it. Grief has its own timetable. You mourn best when you grant grief its natural rhythms and you allow yourself your unique responses.

You are going through a major transition in your life, and by their very nature, life transitions are not easy. Your caregiving is one

49

May I try to tell you again
where your only comfort lies?
It is not in forgetting the happy past.
People bring us well-meant but miserable consolations
when they tell us what time will do to help our grief.
We do not want to lose our grief,
because our grief is bound up with our love
and we could not cease to mourn
without being robbed of our affections.

PHILLIPS BROOKS

part of your present transition—it's the beginning. Something else will follow. The time will come when you will need to give up your caregiving role, so others can focus their attention on you, and so you can allow your relationship with the one you love to evolve and change form.

When your present work is done, you'll have other work to do. You'll have more feelings to experience, some of which you'll be familiar with, others of which may be new. Your strength will be challenged again. Your determination will be tested. Your ability to adapt will be called upon one more time. You will not be given much chance to rest in between. But you will have this advantage: by then you will be more practiced. What you're now going through will condition you. What you're learning in this moment will season you. Rather than a beginner, you'll be a veteran. ◪

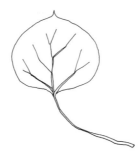

All human wisdom is summed up in two words:
wait and hope.
ALEXANDRE DUMAS

We should not moor a ship with one anchor,
or our life with one hope.
EPICTETUS

"Hope" is the thing with feathers—
That perches in the soul—
And sings the tune without the words—
And never stops—at all—
EMILY DICKINSON

12

For all the turmoil and sadness, you still have reason to hope.

Some days you may wonder if there's anything to look forward to. Burdened by your tiredness or heaviness or loneliness, you may feel you have little to hope for. This may be happening to you right now. If it is, you're not alone. Many caregivers before you have reported similar feelings. But most of these same people have learned that all is not as bleak as it may seem. They would assure you, based on their own experiences, that you still have reason to hope.

• *You can hold hope for the one you care for.* You can hope for their continued comfort. You can be optimistic they'll use this time in positive ways, whether that means resolving the past or enjoying the present, finishing crucial projects or starting new ones, drawing close to others or drawing close to the Supreme Other. You can watch for those signs they're growing and healing emotionally and spiritually. You can hope that, within the limits their illness imposes, they will live richly and fully until it's their time to die. And that when that time comes, they will be ready. And that when they go, they will go in peace.

• *You can hold hope for yourself.* You can hang on to the belief that you'll keep doing the best you can under these pressing circumstances, knowing no one can ask for more. You can trust you'll find resilience and strength when you need it, acceptance and understanding when you wish it, assistance and companionship when you yearn for it. You can have faith you'll mature as a result of this experience, growing more compassionate and more open. You can choose to believe the price you're paying for your love and your growth will one day seem worth it.

If you do not hope,
you will not find what is beyond your hopes.

CLEMENT OF ALEXANDRIA

To be a traveler on this earth,
you must know how to die and come to life again.

JOHANN WOLFGANG VON GOETHE

And shall it be said that
my eve was in truth my dawn?

KAHLIL GIBRAN

You can hope the grieving you're doing today will help you as you grieve tomorrow. You can trust that as you prepare for your loved one's death, you will become better prepared for other deaths that will surely visit you, including your own. You can further pray that this preparation will influence how you *live* as well as how you die. And through it all, you can harbor the hope you'll find a serenity that will ground you, a grace that will free you, and an assurance that will never leave you.

• *You can hold hope for everyone.* Wherever there has been separation, you can hope for connection to grow. Wherever there has been fear, for trust to appear. Wherever there has been despair, for dreams to be born again. You can make it your wish that your family and other families will rise to the occasion that awaits, that friends will do whatever they can to help, and that all the professionals involved will be that and more. You can hope for a sense of community to develop, and for a wonderful celebration of life to emerge, and for one life in particular to be affirmed and lifted up.

You can believe that because of what all of you do together, death will begin to lose some of its sting. Then when you say your final good-byes, you will discover they're followed by glorious hellos, both in time and beyond time. As you surrender to your losses, you will discover they're not without their gains. And finally, as you walk softly and bravely with your loved one as far as you can toward that distant horizon, you will know beyond all doubt that this journey has a name. Its name is love. ▟

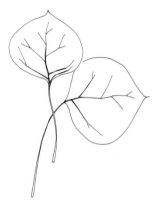

The best things are the nearest:
breath in your nostrils, light in your eyes,
flowers at your feet, duties at your hand,
the path of God just before you.
Then do not grasp at the stars,
but do life's plain, common work as it comes,
certain that daily duties and daily bread
are the sweetest things in life.

ROBERT LOUIS STEVENSON

A Final Word

You probably never gave much thought to the possibility you'd be doing what you're now doing. You probably didn't see yourself caring for the person you love as they prepare to die. But that's now one of your tasks. If you're like most caregivers, you wish you didn't have to learn what you're now learning. You wish life could be the way it once was. You wish death were not so insistent. You wish you had more say in this whole matter. But you don't.

There is much to dislike about this time, much to be fearful of and worry over. There is much that can cause you pain. Consequently, you may wonder if there is anything that can be at all positive about this experience. I believe there is.

• *You may feel as if you're alone, and in some ways you are—but in some very important ways you're also accompanied.* Many others have cared for someone who is dying before you, and their spirit is now with you. Others are caring for loved ones as they die at the same moment you are, and you're united by what you're each doing. You are not the only person to care for this one you love. Professionals are standing by with their unique kinds of help. People who know you, and sometimes even those who don't, will step forward if you ask or if you let them. Others can be with you even from a distance.

• *You may feel this is a painful time, and it is—but there is more to be experienced than just pain.* You can also experience genuine closeness. You can go deeper in your love for one another. You can strengthen your ties with those around you, and you can be strengthened by the same ties. You can discover joy in unexpected places. You can know laughter at unexpected times. It's possible to come upon a sense of peace that grounds you when you need it most.

Look to this day,
for it is life, the very life of life.
In its brief course lie all the verities and
realities of existence:
the bliss of growth,
the glory of action,
the splendor of beauty.
For yesterday is but a dream,
and tomorrow is only a vision.
But every today well-lived
makes every yesterday a dream of happiness
and every tomorrow a vision of hope.
Look well, therefore, to this day.
Such is the salutation of the dawn.

FROM THE SANSKRIT

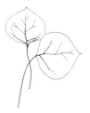

• *You may think you're entering a time of decline, and you are—but decline is only one part of what's happening.* Disease necessarily takes its toll and bodies will all eventually weaken. But an opposite movement can also occur. At the very same time, one's spirit can rise. One's thoughts can build. One's heart can heal. One's love can grow. That's true for the one who's dying, and it's just as true for you.

• *You may think you're restricted by serious limitations, and that's true—but this can also be a time of unusual freedom.* You can choose to let go of the unimportant. You can leave behind the unhealthy. You can release any pettiness. You can stop running away and start really connecting. You can quietly refuse to live someone else's life and proceed to live your own.

• *You may think you're helpless to change what is happening now, and in certain ways you are—but that doesn't mean you're completely powerless.* You can still exert your influence in various ways, and you can make a difference in people's lives. You can see that the one you love receives good care and in proper amounts. You can let others know what you need. You can tell them what helps and what doesn't. You can take charge of your own life in those ways you're able, including the things you say to yourself, which so easily affect your attitude. You can also do something else: you can open yourself to the powerful lessons that come only after you submit to that which is clearly beyond your control.

• *You may experience this as a time of losing, and it is—but loss can have unexpected effects on your life.* You may lose your innocence and gain more wisdom. You may lose what you couldn't imagine living without and gain a strength you never realized you possessed. You may lose some part of your future and regain your present moments. You may lose some portion of yourself and begin to find the whole of yourself.

• *You may see this as an unfortunate interlude in your life, and in some important ways that's true—but that's not the entire story.* This

59

Lord, make me an instrument of thy peace.
Where there is hatred, let me sow love;
where there is injury, pardon;
where there is doubt, faith;
where there is despair, hope;
where there is darkness, light;
and where there is sadness, joy.
Divine Master, grant that I may not so much
seek to be consoled as to console;
to be understood as to understand;
to be loved as to love.
For it is in giving that we receive,
it is in forgiving that we are forgiven,
and it is in dying that we are born to eternal life.

PRAYER OF ST. FRANCIS

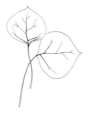

time can be more than a misfortune. In the midst of all that is ordinary about these days, sacredness can sometimes break through, and with surprising effects. In the middle of all that you don't understand about these events, you can sometimes catch a glimmer of a larger vision and a greater purpose.

Through this experience of caring for the one you love as they prepare to die, may the words of English writer George Byron hold true for you:

"*Come what may, I have been blessed.*"

Come what may, you have made a difference in someone's days on earth, and they have made a difference in yours. Come what may, you have known life for its fullness and joy for its richness. Come what may, you have touched with love and you have been touched *by* love. Come what may, you have been a blessing, and more than that, you have been blessed. ◩

Additional Resources by James E. Miller

Illness, Dying, and Caregiving

Books

When You Know You're Dying
12 Thoughts to Guide You Through the Days Ahead

When You're Ill or Incapacitated
12 Things to Remember in Times of Sickness, Injury, or Disability
When You're the Caregiver
12 Things to Do If Someone You Care For Is Ill or Incapacitated

The Caregiver's Book
Caring for Another, Caring for Yourself

Welcoming Change
Discovering Hope in Life's Transitions

A Pilgrimage Through Grief
Healing the Soul's Hurt After Loss

Videotapes

The Grit and Grace of Being a Caregiver
Maintaining Your Balance as You Care for Others

Listen to Your Sadness
Finding Hope Again After Despair Invades Your Life

How Do I Go On?
Re-designing Your Future After Crisis Has Changed Your Life

By the Waters of Babylon
A Spiritual Pilgrimage for Those Who Feel Dislocated

The Natural Way of Prayer
Being Free to Express What You Feel Deep Within

You Shall Not Be Overcome
Promises and Prayers for Uncertain Times

Audiotapes

When You're Ill or Incapacitated
12 Things to Remember in Times of Sickness, Injury, or Disability

Loss and Grief

Books

What Will Help Me?
12 Things to Remember When You Have Suffered a Loss
How Can I Help?
12 Things to Do When Someone You Know Suffers a Loss

Winter Grief, Summer Grace: *Returning to Life After a Loved One Dies*

How Will I Get Through the Holidays?
12 Ideas for Those Whose Loved One Has Died

Videotapes

Invincible Summer: *Returning to Life After Someone You Love Has Died*

We Will Remember: *A Meditation for Those Who Live On*

Nothing Is Permanent Except Change
Learning to Manage Transition in Your Life

Audiotapes

The Transforming Potential of Your Grief: *Eight Principles for Renewed Life*

Spirituality

Books

Autumn Wisdom: *Finding Meaning in Life's Later Years*

A Little Book for Preachers: *101 Ideas for Better Sermons*

Videotapes

Gaining a Heart of Wisdom: *Finding Meaning in the Autumn of Your Life*

Common Bushes Afire: *Discovering the Sacred in Our Everyday lives*

Why Yellow? *A Quiet Search for That Which Lies Behind All That Is*

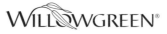

WILLOWGREEN®

P.O. Box 25180 • Fort Wayne, IN 46825 • 219/424-7916

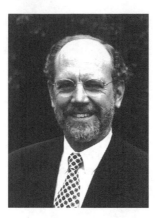

James E. Miller is a clergyman, grief counselor, writer, and photographer who lives and works in Fort Wayne, Indiana. Many of his books, audiotapes, and videotapes deal with illness, caregiving, loss, and grief, but his writing and photography also incorporate the topics of managing transition, healthy older age, and spirituality. He lectures and leads workshops widely, often utilizing his personal photography to illustrate his ideas. He is married to Bernie and together they have three children.

For information about his other resources, including quantity purchases, as well as about scheduling him for a speaking engagement or workshop, contact

Willowgreen
P.O. Box 25180
Fort Wayne, IN 46825
219/424-7916
jmiller@willowgreen.com